Girl Puberty
How to Talk about Puberty and Sex with your Tween Girl

Cath Hakanson

Thanks for buying
Girl Puberty:
How to Talk about Puberty and Sex with your TWEEN
GIRL

As a special Thank You,
you can download your FREE parent guide:

30 of the most common questions kids ask about
puberty (and answers that will make you a badass
mom)

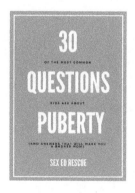

To get it, visit:
https://sexedrescue.com/gp/

ADVANCE PRAISE FOR GIRL PUBERTY

"In *Girl Puberty* Cath Hakanson has written a pitch-perfect conversational book, loaded with information and advice for parents and carers as they guide girls through the physical, emotional and social whirl of puberty. Cath's years of experience and down-to-earth style will boost parents and carers confidence and enable them to support girls with respectful, timely and appropriate guidance and conversations. Highly recommended!"

Jane Bennett, author of *A Blessing Not A Curse and Girltopia*, founder of A Celebration Day for Girls, Mense-Ed and the Chalice Foundation

"One of the difficulties today is to distinguish who is who on the internet and when it comes to talking about sex, you cannot get someone more prepared, committed, knowledgeable or professional than Cath. I would encourage any parent who wants to talk to their kids about puberty to read and use Cath's work as it provides simple, practical and important information to make the conversation as natural as any other talk parents have with their children."

Dr Madalena Grobbelaar, Clinical Psychologist, Psychosexual Therapist & Academic at Women Sexuality Australia

"Cath has created the perfect book for busy parents. Talking about sexuality and relationships can be tricky for most parents – many would rather clean the oven, weed the garden or de-flea the dog, than talk openly and honestly about sex! To this book, Cath has brought her vast experience, wisdom and laugh-a-minute humour."

Dr Lorel Mayberry,
Sexologist and Consultant in Sexuality and Relationship Education,
Department of Sexology, School of Public Health,
Curtin University l President - Borderless Friendship WA Inc

"The book I wish my mother had read, or at least left lying around! This book has all the finer details to answer the questions I know the basics for. As a mother of 3, and teacher, it's a great resource for age appropriate information."

Ren, mum to 14, 13 and 10 yo question askers

"Cath's book is 'puberty in a nutshell' for me and a goldmine of information. I wasn't expecting such a wall of resistance from my daughter. Total denial with fingers in her ears singing la la la la!! But I knew I had to be ready (even though she wasn't) to take advantage of those elusive teachable moments! And I was! Thanks to the clear concise language used and the deep knowledge of puberty in this book.

It's been a long time since my own puberty, and my daughter, while similar, has her own body clock & timetable. So after reading this book, I had a lot more confidence. I can now recognise the range of signs and be there ready with the facts for each situation. Even to the point when I had that first voluntary question from my daughter recently! And we had a great natural conversation! So the moral to this book for me is...you can be ready even if they aren't!! Thanks a million Cath."

Fiona, mother of a 12 year old girl

"As an educator and parent, I think every parent should read this book before puberty hits! It is both concise and comprehensive: Cath doesn't leave anything out but gives us just enough of what we need for every aspect of talking to our kids about puberty. It is a practical step-by-step guide as well as a handy reference, and it even leaves room for a family's cultural and religious beliefs. This is a straightforward yet compassionate handling of a must-have conversation with our kids."

Cory Peppler, teacher, father,
and founder of ParentingDigital.com

"Cath has such a brilliant way of taking the confusion and awkwardness out of those conversations that can have any of us wondering how to start and what to say. Her simple, no-nonsense wisdom makes this book a must-have for every parent.

The conversations we have with our kids are strengthening and life-giving, but some of the important ones can be a little awkward. Cath offers practical wisdom on how to talk to kids about sex and puberty in ways that will help to relieve the 'awkward' (for them and for you!) and open the communication between you and your child or teen on these essential conversations."

Karen Young, Psychologist, author of *Hey Warrior*
and founder of Hey Sigmund

Girl Puberty by Cath Hakanson helps parents of tweens take that first, giant step onto the often bumpy road towards puberty. *Girl Puberty* is a refreshing mix of facts and fun and information for adults looking for the right thing to say and the best way to say it. Puberty can be a roller coaster ride for everyone in the family, and to be armed with the knowledge and skills to negotiate the ride and arrive intact at the other end is exactly what parents and carers need.

Buy the book, read it and study the diagrams before you start to see the body changes and experience the social and emotional whirlwind of puberty. You'll be glad that you did – and so will your girl.

Margie Buttriss, HUSHeducation

"As a parent of a tween, I realised that after reading *Girl Puberty*, there is so much more information I can use to support my daughter during this pubescent stage. Cath Hakanson takes some difficult concepts and explains them in an easy, informative read. *Girl Puberty* covers those dreaded conversations. It gives parents a guide, a puberty manual to feel safe and excited while empowering their child to embrace the changes that are inevitable. I highly recommend this educational read for every parent. The visual explanations are simple and entertaining too!"

Michelle Avichzer, Parent, Teacher, Kinesiologist

Girl

PUBERTY

How to Talk about Puberty and Sex
with your
TWEEN GIRL

CATH HAKANSON

Girl Puberty: How to Talk About Puberty and Sex With Your Tween Girl by Cath Hakanson

Published by Sex Ed Rescue

PO Box 7903

Cloisters Square WA 6000

Australia

sexedrescue.com

For permission contact:

cath@sexedrescue.com

ISBN-13: 978-0-6481089-2-4

**National Library of Australia
Cataloguing-in-Publication entry(pbk)**

Creator: Hakanson, Cath, author.

Title: Girl puberty : how to talk about puberty and sex with your tween girl / by Cath Hakanson.

ISBN: 9780648108924 (paperback)

Subjects: Puberty.

Girls--Health and hygiene.

Girls--Growth.

Table of Contents

Introduction

You're already an expert on puberty because you've been through it yourself.

Maybe you've noticed that your daughter is starting to develop breasts or grow hair in new places. Maybe she isn't showing any signs herself, but you've noticed changes in her friends.

Whichever it is, deep down you realize that it's time to have the talk that you probably never had, or had too late, when you were growing up. It's time to prepare your child for what's to come.

If you're like most parents, including me, preparing your daughter for puberty probably isn't something you've ever thought about before. And now you realize how unprepared you are to talk about it. Well, you can relax for a moment, because this book will prepare you for what lies ahead. It will tell you everything you need to know before you talk to your daughter about the changes that will take place in her. This book covers important things, such as what puberty is all about, why it happens, when and how you should start talking, and what you should talk about.

For more than 20 years, I've been helping people get more comfortable with sex. I've answered their questions, listened to their fears, empowered them with the right information, and pointed them in the right direction. After hearing thousands of parents ask me the same questions about puberty over and over again, I've worked out what they want.

Parents want to know how to have honest conversations that will guide their child through puberty and strengthen their relationship without them feeling embarrassed, awkward or nervous.

But they don't know how to start.

This book will help you get started with talking. It will help you to:

- Understand what puberty means for your daughter so you are fully prepared to answer her questions.

- Realize the importance of discussing puberty before it starts so your daughter isn't surprised, confused or frightened.

- Know the evolving changes that happen during puberty, and when they are likely to happen, so you can confidently identify them and prepare your daughter for what comes next.

- Create crucial talking points you can use with your daughter before she gets misinformation from somewhere else, so you have the right information to share at the right time.

- Develop basic tools to help you easily talk to your daughter, even if she is reluctant to talk about puberty.

This book won't just show you how to talk to your daughter about puberty. It will show you how to have the type of relationship where she can talk to you about anything, no matter what. But you need to start talking sooner rather than later, because puberty is on its way, whether you like it or not!

As much as we would all like to leave it for someone else to address (me included), you love your daughter and know that she deserves to hear about the changes that are going to happen to her from you, so that she can turn to you for support, guidance and information.

Empower your daughter with the right information so that when the time comes, she doesn't make the wrong decisions around love, sex and relationships.

Happy talking!

What Is Puberty?

Puberty is going to happen whether you want it to or not, but at least it happens gradually.

Puberty can mean many different things, but, basically, it is when your daughter's body changes from being a child to an adult. It is the last time that her body will grow. Puberty isn't the last time that her body will change though, because, as we know, our bodies will keep on changing for our whole lives. Luckily, puberty doesn't happen overnight. It can take from two-to-five years, up to 10 years for your daughter's body to change. This is a good thing, as it gives her time to get used to the changes that will slowly be happening to her. Puberty is about more than just her body changing. Her relationships with her family, friends and peers will change. Her feelings and even her personality will change too.

What does this all mean?

Puberty means your daughter will soon be fertile, that she can become pregnant and give birth to a baby. And that you could become a grandparent! But does this mean that she is ready to become a parent. Most likely not. Just because her body is capable of reproducing doesn't mean she's necessarily ready to become a parent, but she does need to know that this could happen.

When will puberty happen?

The time puberty starts is different for everyone. It can be earlier for some girls and later for others. Everyone is different. Usually, puberty will start some time between the ages of eight and 15. When your daughter's body is the right size and shape for her, the hormones that start the changes will be triggered, and her body will begin to change. It is important to remember that you can't rush or delay puberty. This can be hard for some girls, especially if they're the first or the last to sprout breasts. They will see themselves as being different from their friends, and will wonder if they are normal.

If she is an early bloomer, your daughter may be teased about her breasts, or attract unwanted attention from her peers. She will most likely be wondering what's wrong with her, as she is the only one whose body is changing. If she's a late bloomer, she may be worried that she hasn't yet started to change, and she will wonder what is wrong with her. It is important that your daughter understands that puberty will happen when her body is ready for it, and that everybody is different.

If you started puberty early, the chances are that your daughter will be an early bloomer. If you started puberty late, your daughter may be a late bloomer too.

When to worry

Some girls start puberty earlier or later than you would expect. An early start to puberty is called precocious puberty. Precocious puberty is defined as the development of breasts before the age of eight, or the start of periods before the age of nine. If this happens to your daughter, you should seek medical advice.

If your daughter does not have any physical signs of puberty by the age of 15 to 16, or periods by the age of 16 to 17, you should seek medical advice as to why puberty is delayed. Usually, puberty is delayed because of a hormonal imbalance, being underweight, or being under extreme stress. Rarely, developmental or chromosomal abnormalities can be found.

What makes puberty happen?

Hormones are responsible for making the changes to your daughter's body during puberty. Hormones are chemicals that all our bodies make. They travel throughout the body in our bloodstream, from the place they are made, to the place they do their work. Their job is to start something working. During puberty, the job of some hormones is to make the body capable of reproducing.

The pituitary gland

During puberty, it all starts because of a gland at the base of the brain known as the pituitary gland. One day, when the body is ready, the brain sends a message to the pituitary gland that tells it to start releasing growth hormones into the bloodstream. The hypothalamus produces a hormone called gonadotrophin-releasing hormone (GnRH). This hormone stimulates the pituitary gland to release two hormones: follicle-stimulating hormone (FSH) and luteinizing hormone (LH). These hormones travel through the blood to the ovaries and trigger the release of estrogen and progesterone.

The pituitary gland is the master gland that tells all other glands what to do. It tells the other glands to start making the hormones that are needed to turn your child into an adult. Hormones are the chemical messages that allow different parts of the body to communicate with each other. Think of it like a telephone line, where everyone's telephones are connected by wire cables, and we can send messages (talk) through the telephone lines. The body has its own telephone lines (bloodstream), where the glands are sending hormones (chemical messages) to the different parts of the body. The pituitary gland sends a message to the ovaries, telling them to start producing the hormones progesterone and estrogen. This causes the egg (ovum) to be released from the ovary.

THE PITUITARY GLAND

THE PITUITARY GLAND SENDS A MESSAGE TO THE OVARIES, TELLING THEM TO START MAKING ESTROGEN AND PROGESTERONE

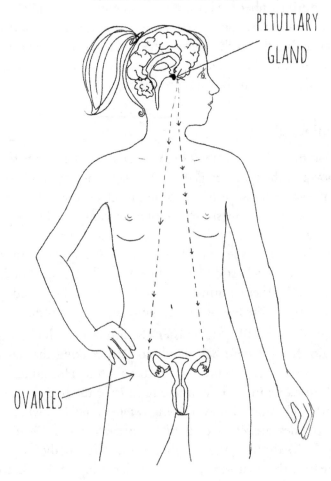

PITUITARY
GLAND

OVARIES

Estrogen and Progesterone

These important hormones have different jobs to do. Estrogen is responsible for the growth of breasts, the changes in body shape such as hips, legs, and breasts, and the development of the reproductive organs. Progesterone and estrogen together prepare the uterus for menstruation or pregnancy.

Ovulation

Your daughter's eggs have been inside her ovaries since she was a fetus growing inside your uterus. Estrogen tells the eggs to mature. It also tells the ovaries to prepare an egg (ovum) for release into the fallopian tubes. The egg will travel along the fallopian tubes and into the uterus. This whole process of ripening an egg for release from the ovary is called ovulation. Ovulation is when the eggs stored in the ovaries begin to ripen, with one being released every four weeks or so, plus or minus a few days.

The ovaries are about the size of a large grape.
An ovum (egg) is the size of a grain of sand.
The uterus is about the size of a pear.

OVULATION

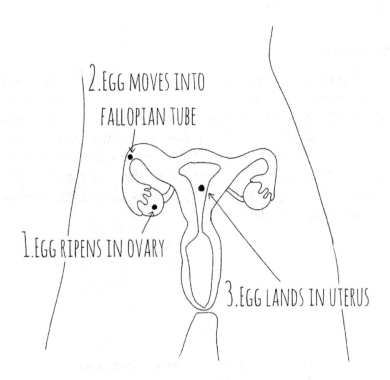

2. EGG MOVES INTO FALLOPIAN TUBE

1. EGG RIPENS IN OVARY

3. EGG LANDS IN UTERUS

Menstruation

While the egg is ripening and getting ready to come out, the lining of the uterus starts to thicken, just in case a sperm joins with the egg, resulting in pregnancy. If the egg is joined with a sperm, the body will begin to prepare itself for pregnancy. If the egg is not joined with a sperm, the lining of the uterus will begin to dissolve. This dissolved lining comes out of the vagina, and is known as a period, menstruation or menstrual blood. Two weeks after the period, another egg is released and the whole process of ovulation begins all over again.

MENSTRUATION

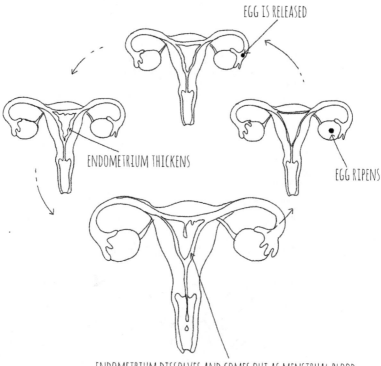

EGG IS RELEASED

ENDOMETRIUM THICKENS

EGG RIPENS

ENDOMETRIUM DISSOLVES AND COMES OUT AS MENSTRUAL BLOOD

Fertilization

This is what happens when the sperm meets the egg. Fertilization usually happens during sexual intercourse, but it can also happen with assistance, for example, with in vitro fertilization (IVF). During sexual intercourse, sperm is released into the vagina when the male ejaculates semen. The sperm will then swim through the vagina and uterus, and up into the fallopian tubes, looking for an egg to fertilize. The egg is fertilized while it is still within the fallopian tube. It will continue travelling along the fallopian tube and into the uterus, where it will attach itself to the thickened uterine lining.

FERTILIZATION

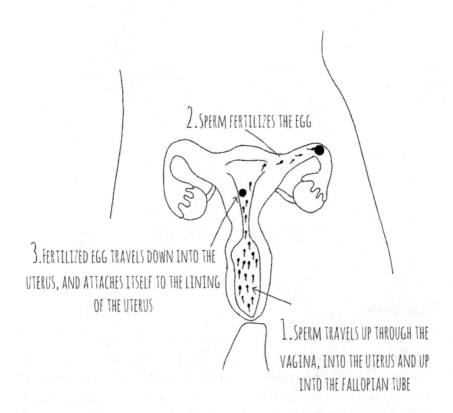

2. SPERM FERTILIZES THE EGG

3. FERTILIZED EGG TRAVELS DOWN INTO THE UTERUS, AND ATTACHES ITSELF TO THE LINING OF THE UTERUS

1. SPERM TRAVELS UP THROUGH THE VAGINA, INTO THE UTERUS AND UP INTO THE FALLOPIAN TUBE

The body parts

When you start talking about puberty, it is important to know the names of the different parts you will be talking about. Below you will find some images and child-friendly definitions your daughter will understand.

Anus: The opening that is below the vulva, where feces (poo) comes out. Boys have an anus too.

Cervix: The opening of the uterus that joins it with the vagina. You can find it deep inside, at the very top of your vagina.

Clitoris: A part that is behind the vulva and wraps around the vagina. The smallest part, about the size of a pea, can be seen outside the body, hidden under a small bump of skin, just above the urethra where the urine (pee) comes out. It can feel good when you touch it.

Fallopian tubes: Special tubes, like cooked spaghetti, that carry the egg from the ovaries to the uterus.

Labia majora: The outer lips that surround the vaginal opening. These are thicker and will eventually be covered in hair on the outside skin.

Labia minora: The inner lips that surround the vaginal opening. These are thinner and will not be covered in hair.

Mons pubis: The soft rounded area that sits above the pubic bone. Eventually, it will be covered in pubic hair.

Ovaries: Special organs that produce the eggs or ova. In girls they are about the size of a grape.

Uterus: A bag made of muscle that in a girl is about the size of a pear. It is the place for a baby to grow, and stretches bigger as the baby grows.

Urethra: A narrow tube that leaves from the bladder and comes out of a small opening in the vulva carrying urine.

Urethral opening: The small opening in the vulva where the urethra comes out of the body. It can be found between the clitoris and the vagina. Boys have a urethral opening too.

Vagina: A stretchy tube that goes from the uterus to the outside of the body. It is the opening that you can feel at the bottom of the vulva.

Vulva: Thick folds of skin that cover the opening to the vagina. There is an outer part which is the labia majora, and an inner part which is the labia minora.

THE INSIDE PARTS (FRONT VIEW)

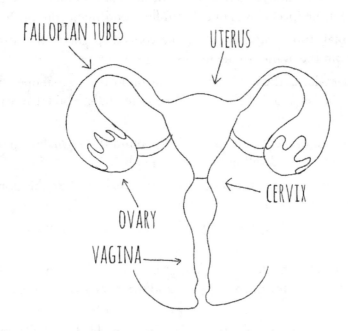

THE INSIDE PARTS (SIDE VIEW)

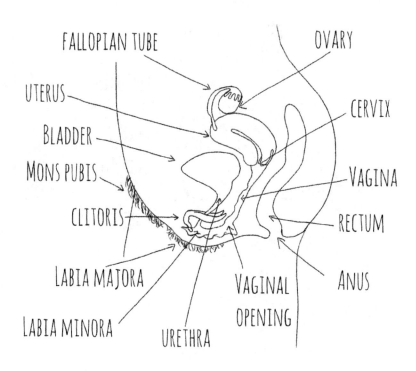

FALLOPIAN TUBE

OVARY

UTERUS

CERVIX

BLADDER

MONS PUBIS

VAGINA

CLITORIS

RECTUM

LABIA MAJORA

ANUS

LABIA MINORA

VAGINAL OPENING

URETHRA

THE OUTSIDE PARTS

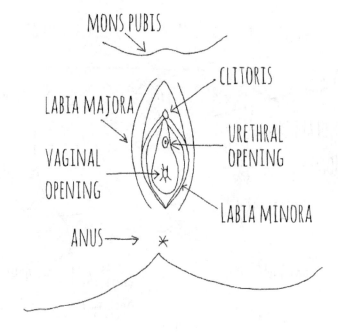

CLITORIS

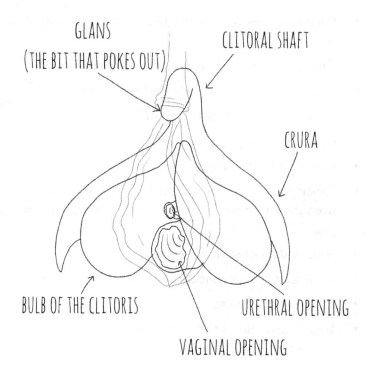

GLANS
(THE BIT THAT POKES OUT)

CLITORAL SHAFT

CRURA

BULB OF THE CLITORIS

URETHRAL OPENING

VAGINAL OPENING

What do kids need to know?

Every girl is different. Some girls will want to know every detail, whereas others will be happy with just the basics. The good thing is you won't be expected to remember all of this, or have to talk about it all. That is where books become invaluable. Books will include all the technical details, which means you don't need to remember everything. A basic understanding will help with answering their questions.

So, what are the main messages we need to give to girls?

- Puberty means your body will change from being a kid to an adult.

- Changes are both physical and emotional.

- Puberty happens to all kids, and it is normal.

- Puberty means you can reproduce.

- Changes are very gradual.

- Puberty happens to boys too!

- Puberty doesn't happen overnight; it takes two-to-five years from start to finish. This gives you time to get used to the new you.

- Some kids start sooner, some start later.

- Some kids change quickly, some kids change more slowly.

- Everyone is different.

- Your body is already programmed to create the body that you are meant to have.

Why You Must Talk About Puberty

*Don't waste this opportunity to be your child's number-one
source for information on love, sex and relationships.*

Reasons for talking to girls about puberty

Sometimes it can feel as if there are more reasons not to talk
than there are to talk. Will you say too much and overwhelm
her? Will you say too little and misinform her? Do girls need
to understand puberty differently than boys? How do you approach
the topic without embarrassing her or yourself? What if your daughter
shows no interest or covers her ears while walking away?

You're not alone if you have already asked yourself some of these
questions, as they are questions that parents commonly ask. If you
have some lingering doubts about whether you're doing the right
thing, you should know that most parents feel the same. Talking to
your daughter about puberty is one of the greatest gifts you can give
her, and yourself.

Here are some of the reasons why you should be talking to her
about puberty sooner rather than later:

Puberty will be much easier for her

Girls who know what to expect during puberty will usually have a much better experience than girls who are unprepared. Think back for a moment to your own memories of puberty. Did your parents talk to you about puberty and tell you what to expect? If they did, you are one of the lucky few! Most of us don't have very good memories of our own journey through puberty. We didn't have parents who spoke to us about puberty. Or if we did, it was usually the one big talk that we didn't really understand, which meant that we had to go through puberty unprepared for what was going to happen to us. So, we know that girls will cope much better with puberty when they know what to expect. They need to know about what changes are going to happen to them, why it is happening, and how to take care of their new body. You aren't alone if you want your daughter to have a much better experience of puberty than the one you had.

She'll hear about puberty anyway

Unless you live in the middle of nowhere with no contact with the outside world, your daughter will eventually hear about puberty. She will hear her friends talk about it at school as they whisper about growing hair down there or about their first trainer bra, or as they giggle and point out the older girls with their newly-developing breasts. She will hear about it in class. Reproduction and the changes that happen to our bodies is in most school curriculums around the world. Don't be surprised if one day she brings a letter home from school advising you about these forthcoming lessons. She may learn about puberty from her favorite TV show, on the internet, or in a book.

Regardless of whether you have talked about puberty or not, your daughter is eventually going to hear about it. The problem is that what she hears will often be negative and inaccurate. This means that it is really important for you, the parent, to be the one who tells her all about puberty. This is your opportunity to provide her with the right information in a way that prepares her instead of scaring her. More importantly, puberty is a great time to start talking to your daughter about what sexual behaviors and attitudes are okay, and not okay, in your family. Your daughter is now reaching the age where she will start forming her own attitudes and beliefs about sexuality. By sharing yours with her, you are providing her with a moral compass to guide her as she makes sense of the mixed messages that she receives from the media, her peers, and the world around her.

Kids want us to talk to them about growing up

Research tells us that 12-to-15-year-olds consistently say their parents are the most important influence when it comes to making decisions about sex, even more than their friends, the media, religious leaders, their brothers or sisters, or their teachers. Parental influence does decline as kids get older, though, which means that it is important to start talking sooner rather than later.[1]

Kids are now shaping their lifelong values

This is the time your daughter will be working out her own thoughts, beliefs and attitudes about the world around her. She will be making important decisions about what attitudes and behaviors are okay, and not okay, when it comes to love, sex and relationships. Which is why it is so important that you are there to guide her. You can't tell your daughter what her values and beliefs will be, you can only guide her. Do you have the exact same values as your parents? Probably not. You may share some of the same values as your parents, but you will also have some that are yours alone. And your siblings will have a completely different set of values, too, despite the fact that you were all influenced by your parents in the same way. The reason that you share some of the same values as your parents is because they influenced you. Some of their values must have made sense, and you took them on board as your own. And some you developed by yourself, influenced by what you saw on TV, heard in music, or learned by talking with your friends and by watching your peers.

Your daughter will be the same. She will make up her own set of values but she will listen to what you say. If you don't share your values with your daughter, you can't expect to have any influence on what sexual attitudes and behaviors she develops. If you want to have

1 The National Campaign to Prevent Teen and Unplanned Pregnancy. (2016). Survey Says: Parent Power Washington, DC: Author.

any say in it, you will have to talk to her, and explain why you feel the way you do.

A stronger relationship

By having open and honest conversations about it, you can guide your daughter through puberty and strengthen your relationship. As much as you'd like to leave it up to someone such as the school or her friends to address the issue, you love your daughter and know she deserves to hear from you about the changes happening to her. This way, she'll be confident about what comes next, knowing that she can turn to you for support, guidance and information.

Research tells us that it is easier for teens to delay sexual activity and to avoid teen pregnancy when they are able to have open, honest conversations about these topics with their parents. Overall closeness between parent and child, shared activities, parental presence in the home, and parental caring and concern, were all associated with a reduced risk of early sex and teen pregnancy. Teens who are close to their parents and feel supported by them are more likely to delay sex, to have fewer sexual partners, and to use contraception.[2]

You already know a lot about puberty

You have firsthand experience of puberty. You have already been through it and know what it can be like. You know what it is like to find that first hair, the embarrassment of being teased for wearing a bra, or feeling embarrassed as someone you really like walks past and looks at you. Sharing stories from your own journey through puberty helps your daughter know that you have been there, and that you understand what she is going through.

A more confident child

Girls who know what to expect from puberty are going to be a lot more accepting of the changes they will soon be experiencing. They will feel a lot more positive about their bodies and feel good

2 Albert, B. (2012). With One Voice 2012: America's Adults and Teens Sound Off About Teen Pregnancy. Washington, DC: The National Campaign to Prevent Teen and Unplanned Pregnancy.

about being a girl. They will also be a lot more accepting of their own individual differences, and be happy with who they are instead of unhappy about who they aren't! [3] It is helpful for girls to know that what is happening to them is normal, and that it is happening to their friends too.

Good practice for even trickier conversations

The more you talk about tough topics like puberty, the easier it gets. Eventually, you will be able to talk to your daughter without feeling as embarrassed, awkward or nervous. By the time you get around to some of the other tough topics, such as dating and sex, you'll have had a bit of experience, and you will find it a lot easier than if you were starting afresh. There are plenty of good reasons why you should be talking to your daughter about puberty sooner rather than later.

---

3 Goldman, R & Goldman, J. (1988). Show me yours! Understanding children's sexuality. Ringwood. Penguin Books.

When To Start Talking About Puberty

Puberty will start when your body is ready for it. You can't rush it, stop it, or make it slow down!

When is a good time to start talking?

There are a few signs that you can look out for that will let you know.

You should be ready to start talking to your daughter about puberty if:

- She is beginning to develop breasts or grow pubic hair.
- You notice that some of the girls in her grade level are beginning to grow breasts.
- She is between eight-and-12 years old.
- She starts to ask you questions about puberty.

What age should I expect to see changes?

You'll start to see physical changes in your daughter anywhere between the ages of eight and 14, but usually between 10 and 12. Remember, every girl is different. Some girls will be earlier or later than their friends. Some may have their changes in a slightly different order. Every girl is different, and it is usually normal.

When is it too early to talk?

You can start talking to kids about puberty from a very young age. By talking when they are younger, you are gently introducing the concept to them that one day their body will start to change from being a child's body to an adult body. Kids as young as three or four will have no trouble grasping this concept. They won't really understand why, or even want to know, but they will accept it as just another thing that will one day happen to them. They will see puberty as being normal.

There are many possible opportunities for talking about puberty to young children. Your three-year-old might walk into the bathroom when you're changing your tampon or pad. She might ask why you're bleeding down there. Your five-year-old might be upset because her 13-year-old brother won't have a bath with her anymore, and she wants to know why. Your seven-year-old might have noticed that some of the older girls at school are growing breasts and wants to know if this will happen to her too. These are all situations where you can provide your daughter with basic information that will satisfy her curiosity. You don't need to worry about giving her too much information. Anything that she doesn't understand, will be forgotten because it just won't make sense to her.

When is it too late to talk

Sometimes you can wait too long to start talking about puberty, especially if your daughter has already started to menstruate. If this is your situation, it still isn't too late. It is better to be late than to never talk at all. You still have the opportunity to be able to prepare your daughter for what comes next and to let her know that she can turn to you for support, guidance and information.

Can dads talk to daughters about puberty?

There is no reason why fathers can't talk to their daughters about puberty. Some girls are comfortable talking about their changing body with their father, and some girls aren't. Let your daughter be the guide regarding what she is comfortable with. If you get the sense that she isn't comfortable, try to involve a woman that she trusts, such as an aunt, an older cousin, or a family friend.

Whether dads join in the conversations or not, just being there for your daughter is enough. By acknowledging that her body is changing, or by letting her know that you are there for her, you are helping. It could be something as simple as buying her some pads when out shopping, or sharing a story about your own memories of puberty, perhaps buying her a bar of chocolate when she's sitting on the lounge holding a hot water bottle to her tummy. Letting your daughter know that puberty is okay, that you know what happens, that you are proud of her, and you love her, is incredibly helpful.

What Changes Happen During Puberty?

We all go through the same changes. For some, they happen in a different order, sooner or later, faster or slower. But at the end of the day, she'll have a grown-up body.

A time of change

Puberty is that time when your daughter will change from a child to an adult. Luckily these changes happen slowly over a two-to-10-year period, which means that your daughter has plenty of time to get used to her new body. The first changes that happen with puberty are hidden, as they happen on the inside. From around the age of eight, your daughter's body will slowly start to release hormones. It isn't until she is around 11-to-13 years old that you will start to see any changes to the outside of her body. For some girls, they can be as young as eight or nine, or as old as 15. The important thing to remember is that each girl will grow at her own pace, which is the pace that is right for her body.

Changes to her body

There are many visible and invisible changes that will happen during this time. Some of the changes that happen to your daughter's body will be easy to spot, but others won't be, as they are hidden inside her body. Although the timing of puberty can be different for every girl, the sequence of changes that will happen to your daughter is more predictable. It is important to remember, though, that for some girls, it may be different. Most girls will develop breasts first, whereas for others it may be pubic hair. Whichever order it happens, both are completely normal.

Below you will find a rough guide to the changes you can expect and when. Not every girl will follow this pattern, but it will give you an idea of what to expect. Many of the changes during puberty will also overlap each other, and may happen over several years. Remember, every girl is different and almost anything can be normal. If concerned, talk to your family doctor.

Eight to 11 years

Hidden changes

The first changes that will happen to your daughter are hidden as they are happening deep inside her body. The body will start to release hormones that will trigger the changes to start happening. The main hormone for girls is estrogen. It will begin to surge in your daughter's body, making her ovaries grow much larger, but no changes can yet be seen outside her body.

Eight to 14 years
(Average 11 to 12 years)

Breasts

Every girl is different, but the first visible sign of puberty that you will most likely see in your daughter is the development of breasts. A small number of girls can be different and will develop pubic hair before breasts. This is completely normal and nothing to worry about.

Breast development happens slowly, over three-to-five years. Breast buds will develop and your daughter may feel a small lump behind her nipple. The nipples will be tender and elevated, and the area around the nipple, the areola, will increase in size. Breast buds are made up of breast tissue, which, over time, will begin to grow bigger and bigger, developing into a round and full breast.

Pubic hair

Next, your daughter will start to grow a small amount of fine soft hair on the skin around the external genitals, on the mons pubis and the labia majora. Over the next couple of years, her pubic hair will grow thicker and darker. It may be coarse or fine, straight or curly. Every girl is different.

Growth spurt

The next thing to happen is usually a growth spurt. Some girls are different, and may have a growth spurt at either the same time as, or just before, breasts. Regardless of what comes first, your daughter will grow a lot taller over the next two-to-three years, as well as gain weight. Before she grows taller, her feet and hands will usually have a growth spurt of their own.

If you find yourself joking about her going up a shoe size overnight,
then you can be certain that puberty is on its way!

Your daughter's body shape will also begin to change, and she will become rounder and curvier. Her hips will grow wider and she will now begin to show the beginning of a waistline. As her body begins to store fat, she will start to gain weight. Sometimes this weight gain happens quickly, over one-to-two years, or it may happen more slowly over three-to-four years. Some girls worry about the body fat that they gain during puberty, thinking that they need to go on a diet. It is important to remember that your daughter is supposed to gain weight during puberty. The weight and height growth spurts don't always happen at the same time or at the same pace. Sometimes she may feel as if she is getting fat, but then she'll have a growth spurt so the body fat will spread out to fit her new height. If weight gain is rapid, some girls will develop stretch marks. This can be seen as purplish or white lines on the skin. It isn't common but it can happen.

Body odor

It is during puberty that your daughter will now start to sweat. This means that her body odor will change, especially when it comes from her armpits.

Nine to 15 years
(Average 12 to 13 years)

Breasts

Your daughter's breasts will continue to grow, increasing in size and being more cone-shaped and pointy. Her nipple and areola will now be more obvious, becoming larger and darker.

Pubic hair

Her pubic hair will begin to grow coarser and darker, but there still isn't a lot of it. She may also start to grow more hair on her lower legs.

Growth spurt

Her body will still be growing and gaining weight and height.

Reproductive organs

Inside her body, her reproductive organs will grow larger. Her vagina, ovaries, fallopian tubes, and uterus will all grow.

Genitals

Outside her body, her genitals will also begin to change. Her vulva will swell as the different parts begin to grow. Her mons pubis will begin to show a bulge, with the fat pad getting thicker and softer. Her labia majora, the outer lips, will become more fleshy and wrinkly, with their edges beginning to touch or meet up. As the oil glands begin to work, your daughter may notice small, light-colored, slightly-raised bumps on the underside of the skin. Her labia minora, the inner lips, will become more fleshy, wrinkly and more noticeable. Her oil glands will start working, making these tissues moister. They will also darken in color. The clitoris will be larger and more sensitive.

Vaginal discharge

As the vagina grows, your daughter may notice vaginal discharge for the first time. She may notice a white or yellow stain on her underwear, or comment about feeling wet around her vulval area. This is all completely normal and is just the body's way of looking after itself. Some girls worry when this first happens. They think that they may have wet themselves, or that there is something wrong with them. It is important for your daughter to know that she is normal and that her vaginal discharge will change during her menstrual cycle. Sometimes it will be lighter or heavier.

Vaginal discharge is usually the last change that happens before the first period, so she can expect her first period in about six-to-12 months' time. Some girls will start to have vaginal discharge for as long as two-to-three years before their first period. In this case, the discharge will usually become more frequent and in heavier amounts in the last few months leading up to their period.

Menstruation or periods

Some girls may have their first menstrual period.

If your daughter has breasts, some pubic hair and vaginal discharge, you need to prepare her for her period.

10 to 16 years
(Average 13 to 14 years)

Breasts

Her nipple and areola will become more obvious, becoming larger, darker and pointier. Eventually, her breasts will have a fuller, more rounded adult shape. Sometimes breasts grow at different rates, one then the other. They will usually end up a similar size.

Pubic and underarm hair

Her pubic hair will grow thick, curly and become coarser, taking on a more adult triangular pattern of growth. Underarm hair may now start to appear. Some girls may already have underarm hair, but usually, girls start to grow underarm hair one-to-two years after pubic hair.

Growth spurt

Your daughter will continue to grow, and her hips will become rounder, but not at the same rate as before.

Menstruation or periods

If they haven't already started, then the first menstrual period should now start. Most girls start getting their periods about two-to-two-and-a-half years after the start of breasts. Some girls may start just one year later, while other girls start three-to-four years later. Most girls have their first period between the ages of 12 and 13, but some girls start as early as age nine, and others as late as 15.

When your daughter's first period finally does arrive, it is likely to be irregular at first. The timing of her period and the amount of blood loss will vary. For the first few months, or even up to a year, she probably won't ovulate. Once she does start to ovulate, she will then be fertile and capable of becoming pregnant. Some girls ovulate with their first period. If her periods are regular, then there is a good chance that she is ovulating.

Oily skin and hair

We have oil glands all over our bodies, but during puberty, they become a lot more active. Your daughter's skin may become oily, especially around the chin, nose, forehead, chest and/or back. Some girls may develop acne or pimples. Her hair is also more likely to become oily, meaning that she will now need to wash it more frequently.

12 to 19 years
(Average age 15 years)

This is the last stage of changes. Your daughter will now reach her full height and will look like a young adult. She will now be ovulating, which means that her menstrual period will be regular. Her breasts will be fully grown and her pubic hair will have an adult triangular pattern of growth. Her skin will be less oily, which usually means less pimples, except for the occasional one.

Changes to her feelings and relationships

Puberty is not just about getting your daughter's body ready to make babies. It is also about making sure that she is ready to face all the responsibilities that come with being an adult.

While your daughter's body is changing, her brain will be changing too. She will experience changes in:

- The way she feels about herself.
- Her relationship with her parents.
- Her friendships and feelings of love.

33

- What others expect of her.

This is also the time that she will be working out her own thoughts, beliefs and attitudes about the world around her. She will be making important decisions about what attitudes and behaviors are okay, and not okay, when it comes to love, sex and relationships. It is important that you are there to provide your daughter with the support, guidance and information she needs.

Girls who are prepared for puberty are more likely to find it a breeze instead of a hurricane!

Common feelings

Puberty is not necessarily the nightmare that we are all led to believe it is. Every girl is different regarding how she responds to this time in her life. The one thing we do know is that girls who know what to expect from puberty have a much easier time as they go through it. If your daughter has a much easier time, it means that you will too.

Common feelings that your daughter may experience include:

- Struggling with a sense of identity and questions about herself.
- Moodiness, anger and depression.
- Sleeping a bit more than usual.
- Wishing she was older and being in a hurry to grow up.
- A need for more independence and privacy.
- Relationships with her friends and the opinions of others becoming more important than family.
- Being more concerned or worried about how she looks, with a focus on clothes and her body.

- Worrying about what the future holds (school, family, job, etc.).
- Having crushes on actors, singers, teachers, peers, other kids.
- Being curious about changes that are happening to her body, especially her genitals.
- Feeling sexually attracted to people.
- Being more interested in sex than ever before and perhaps fantasizing and masturbating.
- Masturbation taking on a new meaning due to orgasm and sexual feelings.

As you can see, there is a lot happening. What's important is that your daughter understands this is all normal and it happens to everyone. Her friends will be going through the same things too. It is normal for girls to feel anxious about growing up, and to sometimes wonder if they are going crazy. Think back to your own memories of puberty, and you will know what I mean. Puberty is a time of great change and the more support your daughter has, the easier a time it will be for her and ultimately for you too.

Puberty for boys

Boys go through puberty too. Some of their changes are the same, and some of them are very different. Boys usually start puberty about two years later than girls do.

During puberty, changes for boys include:

- Growth spurt – boys grow taller, heavier, more muscular and wider across the shoulders and chest.
- Pimples or acne.
- Voice deepens and the Adam's apple starts to show.
- Oilier hair.
- Hair on arms and legs gets thicker.
- Pubic, underarm, face and chest hair growth.
- Body odor.

- Hands and feet grow bigger and longer.
- Spontaneous erections, ejaculations and wet dreams.
- Penis, testicles and scrotum grow larger.
- Mood changes.

Chapter References

A Blessing Not a Curse: A Mother-Daughter Guide to the Transition from Child to Woman by Jane Bennett. 2002. Sally Milner Publishing Pty Ltd. Bowral.

Adolescence and Puberty. Edited by John Bancroft and June Machover Reinisch. 1990. Oxford University Press. New York.

Gender Differences at Puberty. Edited by Chris Haywood. 2003. Cambridge University Press. Cambridge.

Handbook of Child and Adolescent Sexuality: Developmental and Forensic Psychology. Edited by Daniel S. Bromberg and William T. O'Donohue. 2013. Elsevier. Academic Press. Oxford.

Puberty: Physiology and Abnormalities by Philip Kumanov and Ashok Agarwal. 2016. Springer International Publishing. Switzerland.

What To Talk To Your Daughter About

This is all normal and her friends are going through it too. Soon she will be used to her new body and know how to care for it.

A new self-care regime

Puberty is all about change, and your daughter will soon have a new body to care for. She will need a little bit of advice on how to care for it. Remember, all of this is new to her. What you and I think of as common-sense, such as washing hair more regularly, so it doesn't smell and get oily, isn't as obvious to your daughter. She needs you to slowly start teaching her a whole new regime of self-care, and she will need a fair bit of reminding before she automatically starts to include these new habits into her everyday life.

What to talk about

Relax, you don't need to talk to your daughter about every single thing that is listed below. Let your daughter guide you regarding what is relevant to her. If she is asking about a bra, talk to her about what will happen as her breasts start to grow. Go back to the previous chapter and try to work out where your daughter is regarding the changes to her body. Talk about the changes that are now happening as well as the ones to come.

Just remember, you don't need to talk to your daughter about everything. The fact that you are talking to her is much more important than what you say. By talking about puberty, you're actually letting her know that she can turn to you for support, guidance and information.

Feelings

Your daughter needs to know from the very start that puberty will change her body, but it will also change her feelings as well.

It may help your daughter to know:

- All these new emotions are normal.

- Feeling anxious about growing up is normal. It is normal to not want to grow up or to even be excited or in a hurry to grow up. It can even be normal to feel as if she is going crazy at times.

- Everyone goes through puberty. Some of her friends will be feeling the same things as her. Or different things.

- Going through puberty can be hard.

- There are ways to express intense feelings. She may need some guidance as to what will work for her, such as going for a run or a swim, writing in a journal, or talking to someone.

- Mood swings may happen, where she might feel sad one moment and happy the next. Life for a few years can sometimes be a rollercoaster of changing emotions.

- She may want to spend more time on her own and alone. She needs to know that is okay and that her parents still love her and are still there for her.

- Privacy will become a lot more important and she needs to know her parents will respect her need for more personal space.

- Her brain will be changing and getting ready for her to be an adult. This means that she will want to start making her own decisions about things and to try new things.

- Having sexual feelings is normal and is nothing to feel guilty about. Acting on such feelings, however, is a big responsibility.

For advice on understanding puberty for girls, the book *Untangled* by Lisa Damour is excellent. It will give you insight into what is happening to your daughter psychologically and how to cope as a parent.

Skin care

Your daughter's skin will now become oily, as her oil glands become more active. The oil glands below the surface of her skin will enlarge and start to make sebum, a white oily substance that keeps the skin moist. Sometimes the sebum gets blocked in the oil glands, which means whiteheads or blackheads appear, and if there is infection, then pimples will appear. This means that she'll have oilier skin, sometimes with acne.

As you start to notice her skin becoming oily, it may help your daughter to know:

- She needs to wash her face each day.
- She shouldn't pick at or squeeze pimples (risk of infection and scarring).
- If she is going to wear make-up, it needs to be as natural as possible (oil-based makeup will clog her skin pores).
- Sometimes acne can become severe, and if that happens, you can visit your family doctor for treatment.

How much acne will your daughter have? Chances are that she will have the same amount that you and her other parent had. So, if you didn't have much acne, chances are that your daughter won't either.

Body odor

Your daughter will now start to sweat more and develop body odor for the first time. Sweat glands can be found under her arms, on the palms of her hands, at the bottom of her feet and around her vulva (between her legs). During puberty, these sweat glands become more active, and due to the bacteria on her skin, she will start to develop body odor or BO. This means that at times, she'll stink!

As you start to notice her body smelling, it may help your daughter to know:

- She needs to shower each day.
- She needs to use deodorant or antiperspirant on clean armpits (it doesn't work as well on smelly armpits).
- She may need to look for aluminum-free deodorant (aluminum is linked with breast cancer and Alzheimer's disease).
- She will need to wear clean underwear each day.
- She may need to wash her sports shoes or wear cotton/wool/dry-wicking socks if her feet start to smell.
- She shouldn't use vaginal deodorant sprays as they can irritate her vulva.
- Everyone sweats, so she isn't alone.

Oily Hair

The oil glands that make your daughter's skin oilier are the same ones that will now may make her hair oilier. Each strand of hair has its own oil gland, which keeps the hair shiny and waterproof. During puberty, extra oil is produced, which then makes the hair on her head oily. This means that she'll have hair that may look too shiny, oily and greasy.

As you start to notice her hair smelling or looking oily, it may help your daughter to know:

- She needs to wash her hair more often, possibly daily or every second day.
- She may need to use a special shampoo for oily hair.
- She may need to look for hair styling products that are oil-free or greaseless.

Body hair

As your daughter goes through puberty, she will start to grow hair in some new places. Pubic hair (hair on her vulva) usually happens first, but for some girls, underarm hair grows first. Every girl is different and both are normal. Depending on your cultural background, your daughter may grow hair in some other places too. Some girls will grow hair on their upper lip, their chin or on the side of their face. Or they may grow hair around their nipple and on or between their breasts. If women on either side of your daughter's family have hair in these places, there is a good chance that your daughter will too. If your daughter grows hair in these other places, and there is no family history for this, you should probably see your family doctor, as it needs to be investigated.

The arrival of body hair means you'll need to make a decision about what your family rules are about body hair.

- Can your daughter remove any of her body hair?
- If yes, from what age?
- Which body hair can she remove?
- How can she remove her body hair? Shaving, waxing, or any of the other methods?

As you start to notice new body hair, it may help your daughter to know:

- She will grow hair on her vulva and underarms. It will start off

41

fine and soft, and over the next couple of years, her pubic hair will grow thicker and darker. It may be coarse or fine, straight or curly. Every girl is different.

- She will grow more hair on her arms and legs, and it may be darker in color. This hair may lighten as she becomes an adult but it may not.
- The amount of hair that grows is different for everyone.
- What your family rules are for the removal of body hair. Be prepared for the fact that she may have her own ideas about this.
- Some girls like to remove their body hair. She may experience peer group pressure to shave her legs or armpits. She may want to remove her body hair because she thinks it will make her look and feel more grown up. Talk about the attitudes of your community or culture regarding body hair (many societies feel that women shouldn't have body hair).
- She needs to know about the consequences of hair removal. Once removed, hair will grow back darker.
- Every girl is different. Some girls will have more body hair than others.

Breasts

For most girls, breasts will be the first change they notice. For some girls, their first change will be pubic hair, or even underarm hair. Whichever is first, breasts or hair, both are normal. Breasts grow slowly over a few years before they are fully grown. Most girls will start growing breasts when they are between 10 and 11, but some can start when they are as young as eight or as old as 13.

If you were a late bloomer, chances are your daughter will be too!

It is the hormone estrogen that tells your body to grow breasts. Breasts will start off as breast buds, where a small lump will begin to grow behind the nipple. These buds are made of breast tissue which over time, begin to grow bigger and bigger, developing into a round and full breast.

Luckily, breasts grow slowly over three-to-five years, which means your daughter has plenty of time to get used to them.

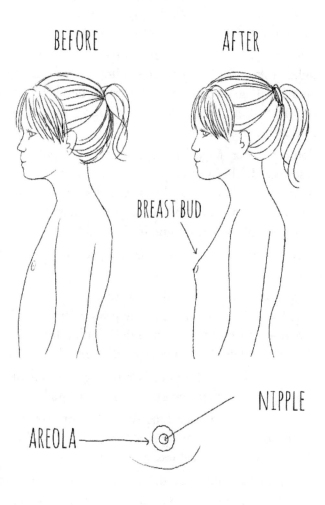

BREAST BUDDING

BEFORE

AFTER

BREAST BUD

NIPPLE

AREOLA

As you start to notice breast buds, it may help your daughter to know:

- Breast buds will develop and she may feel a small lump behind her nipple. The nipples will be tender and elevated, and the area around the nipple, the areola, will increase a little in size.

- Her breasts will grow, swell and hurt just a bit. They may feel itchy as the skin stretches with the new growth.

- They may look pointy or lumpy while they are growing. They will become more round and full once they are fully grown. Breasts come in different shapes and sizes. Hers may look completely different from what she expects.

- The color of her areola will change from purplish to grey to light pink to dark brown depending on your skin color. The areola will get bigger and darker as her breast grows. Her nipples will also start to poke out more and be much more noticeable over time.

- Some girls may have discharge from their nipples, if the nipple is squeezed. This is usually normal and the fluid is made by the body to keep the breast ducts clear. If she keeps on squeezing her breasts, she might make her breasts start producing more, so she shouldn't keep doing it.

- Breasts can feel tender and sore, especially when her body is getting ready for her period.

- They may not grow evenly or at the same rate or to the same size. Sometimes one breast may grow more quickly than the other, which means that she might look a little lopsided. But they are usually the same size by the time they finish growing.

- By the time her breasts stop growing, one breast is usually slightly smaller than the other. This is normal.

- She may feel self-conscious when her breasts first begin to grow. Sometimes wearing a tank top or trainer bra or a loose shirt can make her feel less shy or embarrassed.

- She will eventually need to wear a bra for breast support.

- Every girl is different. Some girls will start to grow breasts sooner or later than their friends, some girls will grow their breasts faster or slower than their friends, and some girls will grow larger or smaller breasts than their friends. Every girl is different!

- Her body will start to grow breasts when it is ready. You can't rush breasts! They will grow at the right time.
- Some girls will feel excited or embarrassed about growing breasts. How does she feel?
- Some people will make comments about her changing body. Sometimes these comments are nice or they can be teasing or even mean. How do you think she'll manage this? What can she do if this happens to her? Who can she talk to?
- Some girls are unhappy with their breast size. She shouldn't let her breast size affect how she feels about herself.
- Her friends are going through the same thing!

Body size and shape

Your daughter needs to know that she will be having two types of growth spurts. She will grow taller and she will also start to get heavier as her body builds muscle and stores fat.

As you start to notice her body shape and size changing, it may help your daughter to know:

- Her hips will broaden, her breasts will get bigger, she will gain weight and grow taller.
- She may feel self-conscious about her new shape, size and fat.
- She may have some growing pains while this happens. The cause is unknown but she may feel it in the legs (calf, front of thigh or behind knees). It may be worse in the afternoon or evening and may waken her during the night. Massage, heat packs and mild analgesia can help.
- She will gain weight and this is what her body is supposed to do. Her body is going to start building muscle and storing fat.
- She may develop stretch marks as her body grows quickly. These will eventually fade over time.

- At times, she may feel fat. This is normal and when her body has its next growth spurt for height, any extra fat will usually spread out. We all have different body shapes, and you can't change the body shape that you are meant to have.
- She doesn't need to worry about dieting. As long as she has a healthy well-balanced diet and enough exercise, her body will do what it is meant to do.
- There is a wide range of body shapes and sizes.
- Her face will change, becoming longer and narrower than it was before.

Voice changes

Your daughter's voice will deepen slightly during puberty. The chances are that neither of you will even notice it changing, as it will happen slowly over a number of years.

Vaginal discharge

Some girls can find it quite alarming when they first notice vaginal discharge. Your daughter may think she is wetting herself, as she becomes aware of the sensation of fluid coming out of her vagina. Or she may wonder what these white/yellow patches are that she finds on the inside of her underwear. Vaginal discharge is a normal part of puberty. Basically, it is secretions from the lining of the vagina and cervix that will come out through the vagina. Often girls are not even aware that it is coming out, but other times they may feel it as it comes out. Most girls usually find it on their underwear. The amount of discharge, the color, and the texture of it changes during the menstrual cycle. It can range from being clear and slippery like egg white, to being white, and either creamy, or thick and pasty. When it dries, it will look white or yellow. All of this is completely normal and is different for every girl.

Vaginal discharge is usually the last change that happens before the first period, so she can expect her first period in about six-to-12 months' time. Some girls will start to have vaginal discharge for as long as two-to-three years before their first period. In this case, the discharge will usually become more frequent and in heavier amounts in the last few months leading up to her period.

When is a good time to start talking about this with your daughter?

Well, if you have already noticed white/yellow stains on her underwear, or you hear the odd comment from her about feeling wet down below, or if she has started to grow breasts and pubic or underarm hair, then now is a good time to start talking.

It may help your daughter to know:

- She might see and feel a clear or white liquid from her vagina or white/yellowish staining on underwear. This is normal and means that her vagina and cervix is working properly.

- Her vaginal discharge will always change. Some days she will have it and other days she won't. Some days it will be heavier and some days it will be lighter. Sometimes it will feel like egg white and other days it will be thick and pasty.

- Discharge doesn't happen every day, just some days of the menstrual cycle.

- Her vaginal discharge will change when she ovulates, signaling that she is now fertile (it changes to help the sperm to reach the egg).

- Paying attention to her vaginal discharge can help her to better understand her body.

- If it changes color or smells, or she becomes itchy or her skin becomes irritated, it might mean that she has an infection. She should seek medical attention, just in case it is an infection.

- She needs to wash her vulva daily, making sure that she washes around the folds of the labia. She can use a low pH soap and water for this. There is no need for powders or deodorants.

- If the discharge is heavy, and making her pants feel wet, she can wear a panty liner or even period pants (underwear with an inbuilt absorbent lining that won't leak).

- Increased vaginal discharge usually means that her period will start sometime in the next six-to-12 months.

- When toileting, wipe from front to back.

- All girls have vaginal discharge. It is normal.

Periods

All girls want to know when they will get their period. It is a much-anticipated event, and seen by many girls as the sign that they have finally become a woman. Girls will usually have a lot of questions about periods, but their main concern will be about when they will get their first period. They will have a lot of unanswered questions and fears about what periods will mean. And they will hear stories from their peers about the horrible things that can happen when you have your period. The more information your daughter has about periods, the more prepared she will be when her time comes. Below you will find information that will address most of the most common concerns that girls usually have about their periods.

What is menstruation?

It may help your daughter to know:

- Menstruation is when the uterus sheds its lining each month and it comes out of the vagina as blood and endometrial tissue.
- Her period can last between three and seven days.
- It usually happens about once a month.
- It means that girls can become pregnant if they have sexual intercourse.
- Periods stop during pregnancy and return once you've had the baby.

When will she get her period?

It may help your daughter to know:

- Every girl is different – some start earlier, and some start later.
- For some girls, they may be as young as nine or 10.
- Other girls may be 14 or 15.
- Most girls get their period when they are 12 or 13.

- Some signs that will give her a clue about when her period is on its way:

    o   Her breasts have already been growing for about two years.

    o   She's had some pubic and underarm hair for the last four-to-six months.

    o   She's been having some vaginal discharge for the last three months. Some girls can have this up to two-to-three years before their first period. In this case, if it starts to get heavier and more frequent, then that is a sign that her period is on its way.

    o   She may get premenstrual symptoms beforehand, like tummy cramps, back ache, headaches, feeling bloated, slight nausea, tiredness and possibly feel irritable, sad, and/or tense.

    o   Find out when her mum started her period – there is a good chance that she'll start hers at around the same age.

- Every girl is different and her period will start when her body is ready for it.

How will she know when her period has started?

The answer to this question may seem pretty obvious, but it isn't to your inexperienced daughter. Think about it for a moment... her current experiences of blood are when she hurts herself. So she probably has quite a few fears about what it means to have blood come out of her vagina each month. Plus, she will have heard a lot of scary stories about what it is like. It is a good idea to provide her with accurate information so she can work out for herself the difference between fact and fiction.

It may help your daughter to know:

- Some blood will start to come out of her vagina.

- She may notice a bright red or dark brown stain on her pants or when she wipes after going to the toilet. Or she may feel some unusual wetness between her legs.

- The blood doesn't pour out like water from a tap. It comes out slowly in drips and there may be some chunks in it (tissue from the lining of her uterus).

- Her first couple of periods will usually have a very light blood flow.

- As they become more regular, they may get heavier and last longer.

- She will need to wear a menstrual pad to absorb the blood and to stop it from staining her clothes.

- If she is really paranoid about her period starting without her knowing, and showing a stain on her clothes, she can wear period underwear (underwear with an inbuilt absorbent lining that won't leak) or a menstrual pad or liner. Some girls need this extra assurance while they are waiting for their period to start.

How much will she bleed?

It may help your daughter to know:

- It is different for every girl.
- Usually it is about two tablespoons (30 mls or 1 fl oz.).
- Blood often starts off as a rusty color and then gets redder.
- It lightens to a rust color again until it stops.
- The amount of blood can vary from day to day – some days are heavier and some are lighter.

What is the menstrual cycle?

It may help your daughter to know:

- Menstrual cycles start from the first day of bleeding until the day before the next bleed.
- When a girl has her period, she bleeds for a few days, then the bleeding stops.
- She may start to notice some vaginal secretions.

- She ovulates.
- Her vaginal secretions will be very slippery like egg white.
- She then has no secretions.
- She may start to have premenstrual symptoms just before her next period.
- The cycle starts all over again.

How long is the menstrual cycle?

It may help your daughter to know:

- It is different for every girl.
- It can be as short as 21 days or as long as 35 days.
- Periods are often irregular in the beginning because it may take the body a while to adjust to all the changes taking place.
- She may have two periods every month and then nothing for a couple of months. Or it may happen every two-to-three weeks for a cycle or two.
- Sometimes she may even have some spotting of blood for a day or two in the middle of her cycle. This is usually nothing to worry about.
- It can take two-to-three years for her cycle to become regular.

When will she be fertile?

Just because she has started her period, doesn't necessarily mean that your daughter is fertile. Ovulation (release of the egg) and menstruation (the shedding of the uterine lining) initially do not always happen together. Some girls will ovulate with their first period but most girls won't. You will know that your daughter is ovulating when her menstrual cycle develops a regular pattern. It doesn't really matter whether she is ovulating or not. All your daughter needs to know is that she is fertile and she can now become pregnant.

It may help your daughter to know:

- She will only be fertile for a few days each month.

- During her fertile days, she can become pregnant (if she has sexual intercourse).

- Girls are fertile for a few days each cycle from the first period until they stop at menopause. (Keep things simple and don't confuse her by telling her that she may/or may not be ovulating at the beginning. At the end of the day, it doesn't really matter. She just needs to know that she can now become pregnant).

- Boys are fertile all the time, from the first time they ejaculate and for the rest of their lives. (Keep things simple and don't confuse her by telling her that it usually takes boys a few years to have enough sperm to help make a baby. She just needs to know that boys are fertile once they start to ejaculate).

What is ovulation?

It may help your daughter to know:

- Ovulation is the periodic release of a mature egg from her ovary.

- This usually happens around the middle of a woman's menstrual cycle.

- Her vaginal secretions will change when she ovulates and become like an egg-white texture.

Could she become pregnant during her period?

It is unlikely, because fertile days are usually around the middle of the menstrual cycle. But, if she has a very short menstrual cycle or bleeds for more days than average, it is possible that she could become pregnant during her period.

It may help your daughter to know:

- It is highly unlikely but it is possible.

- When she is sexually active, she can then learn more about the signals that the body gives when it is fertile.

What is menopause?

It may help your daughter to know:

- Menopause is the stage in life when a woman's menstrual cycle stops.
- It ends because the hormones that cause the eggs to mature in the ovaries stop being produced.
- Menopause usually happens when women are in their late 40s or early 50s.
- Sometimes it can happen earlier, at around 35, or later, in the late 50s.

How do periods make you feel?

It may help your daughter to know:

- Sometimes she may feel different around the time of her period.
- It is different for every girl – some girls feel no different.
- Physical changes may include:
  - o Cramps, pain, bloating, weight gain, food cravings, swollen or sore breasts, swollen hands or feet, skin problems, headaches, dizziness, or irritability.
  - o Cramps and pain usually don't happen for the first few years of having periods. Some girls don't get cramps at all.
- Emotional changes may include:
  - o Short temper, aggression, anger, anxiety or panic, confusion, lack of concentration, nervous tension, fatigue, or depression.
- These physical and emotional symptoms are often called premenstrual syndrome or PMS.
- PMS is related to changes in the body's hormones. As hormone levels rise and fall during her menstrual cycle, they can affect the way she feels, both physically and emotionally.

- There are things that she can do to make herself feel better.
- For PMS, she can:
  - Get plenty of exercise.
  - Eat a healthy diet.
  - Get plenty of sleep.
  - Slow down and have some quiet time.
  - Avoid caffeine.
  - Take natural remedies – ask your pharmacist or visit your local health food shop for advice.
- For period pain and cramps, she can:
  - Just put up with it or try to distract herself.
  - Use a hot water bottle or a heat pack on the tummy.
  - Take a hot bath or shower.
  - Try some gentle exercise.
  - Drink lots of fluids.
  - Ask the local pharmacist about what they recommend for pain relief.

Period celebration

Some families like to celebrate the first period, to acknowledge that their daughter is on her way to becoming a woman. It can especially help your daughter to acknowledge that she is leaving her childhood behind. A celebration of her period is something that you may want to consider in your family. There are lots of different ways that you can do this, but you do need to make sure that it is something that your daughter is happy about. Listen to what she wants to do to celebrate.

Some ideas could include:

- Taking a day off from school and spending it with Mom.
- Going out for dinner as a family.
- Going out for lunch with just your daughter.
- Buying her flowers, chocolates or a card.

- Writing her a letter and telling her about your hopes and dreams for her.

- Putting together a celebration box filled with things she may need during her period, such as period products, new underwear, a heat pack, essential oils, chocolate, etc.

- Giving her a new journal to write in.

- Planting a tree together in the garden.

- Making her something special, such as a patchwork quilt or a piece of embroidery.

- Giving her tickets to a new play, music concert or movie.

- Having a sleepover with friends.

- Buying a keepsake gift or memento.

- Taking her shopping to buy a new outfit.

You could also look at attending a one-day workshop with your daughter. A Celebration Day for Girls is a one-day workshop for 10-12 years old girls with their mother or a female carer. It was designed by Jane Bennett to support girls and mothers at this special threshold in both their lives, and to provide an affirming, grounded and connected celebration of the journey to womanhood. These workshops are offered worldwide and you can find more information here - Celebration Day for Girls. (http://celebrationdayforgirls.com/)

There are lots of different things that you can do to celebrate with your daughter. The main thing is that it is something she wants to do.

Remember, what matters to your daughter is the fact that you are acknowledging her transition and that you are spending time just with her.

Period products

There are a lot of different period products out there: pads, tampons, menstrual cups and sea sponges. You can go natural with reusable cloth products, or you can just buy disposable products at the supermarket. It is pretty much a personal choice as to what your daughter will want to use.

The easiest thing to start with is pads. Your daughter needs to be comfortable with inserting her finger into her vagina before she will be ready to use a tampon. Unless your daughter is a gymnast or a swimmer, keep it simple and start off with pads. You will need to have a supply of pads on hand. There is a wide choice of pads available to use. You can find products that are specifically targeted for girls or teens. Just look for the packaging that looks brighter or more juvenile.

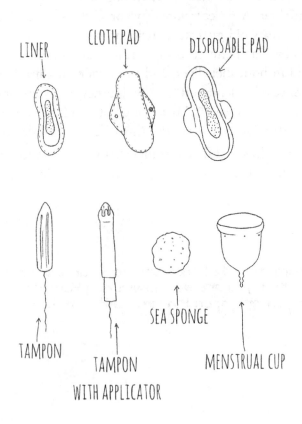

PERIOD PRODUCTS

LINER

CLOTH PAD

DISPOSABLE PAD

TAMPON

TAMPON
WITH APPLICATOR

SEA SPONGE

MENSTRUAL CUP

Period starter kits

You can google 'period starter kit' and you will find lots of companies that have free samples they will send to you. This is worth doing as you can then look at the different products and try them before you buy them. It is a good idea to do this early, so your daughter has more time to get used to these products.

Period kit

A period kit is basically a discreet bag that holds the essentials for having her period. She will then keep it in her schoolbag to use when she has her period.

A period kit can contain:

- Two or three pads.
- Spare underwear in case of leaks.
- Plastic bags to hold stained underpants, or to put used pads in if there isn't a bin handy.
- Cleansing wipes or hand cleanser, just in case she needs to clean blood off her hands before leaving the toilet cubicle.

There is a lot more that you can include, but you need to remember that it needs to be small and compact. Girls are easily embarrassed at this age, so they will want something that is discreet rather than too obvious. They don't want one of the boys to see it and shout, 'Hey, guess who's got her period today!'. A pencil case is ideal as it will blend in with her school gear.

If your daughter is reluctant to have a period kit, remind her that it may come in handy for her friends too, in case they ever get caught without a pad. A good time to make up a period kit is when your daughter is 12, or earlier if she has started to show some signs of puberty. It is never too early for a period kit, and it can just disappear into her schoolbag.

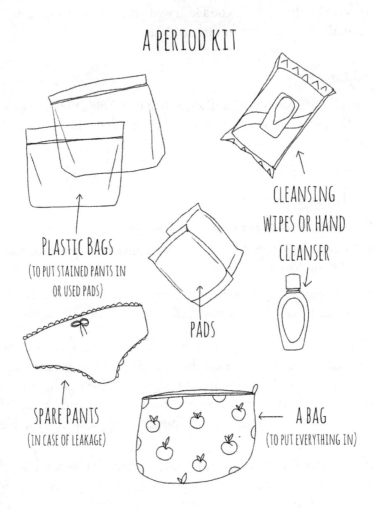

A PERIOD KIT

PLASTIC BAGS
(TO PUT STAINED PANTS IN
OR USED PADS)

CLEANSING
WIPES OR HAND
CLEANSER

PADS

SPARE PANTS
(IN CASE OF LEAKAGE)

A BAG
(TO PUT EVERYTHING IN)

Pad practice

The best way to get your daughter comfortable with menstrual products is to let her play with them. The best time to do this, of course, is before her first period. But you don't want to start too early. Your daughter will most likely forget everything you talk about, or be overwhelmed by all the information you'll share with her.

Your daughter is ready for this activity if she has started to grow breasts, has pubic or underarm hair and/or is 12-to-13 years old.

The best way to practice with pads is to find an afternoon together where it is just the two of you. I know that this can sometimes be impossible, especially if you have other kids, but your daughter will be much more receptive to this activity if she knows that it is just her and Mom, without the distraction of others.

If you are a dad and don't have a mom available, you can still do this activity. You could find an auntie, a female friend or an older girl cousin who can chat with your daughter. It needs to be someone she likes and respects. Or you could be upfront with her, acknowledge that you don't know much about this pad thing either, but you're willing to learn, if she is okay with it. You'll need a supply of different menstrual products – pads, liners and tampons. You can buy a selection of different products or order a period starter kit.

Then one afternoon, when it is just the two of you, get them out and play. You could:

- Unpack some pads and compare the sizes and thicknesses of them.
- Explain why you would wear one type of pad over the other.
- Tip some liquid onto the pad and see what happens.

- Peel the paper strip off the pads and apply them to her underwear. Show her how you can place it in her underwear with the sticky side down. Talk about the best style of underwear to wear (firm not loose fitting).

- Practice sitting on the toilet and putting a pad in. Try showing or explaining how you do it.

- Show her how to roll up a used pad for disposal. Talk about how she can't flush pads down the toilet as it will block the toilet and it could overflow.

- Discuss suitable places for the disposal of used products at home.

- Talk about the special bins that you often find in toilets and explain that they are for this purpose. Discuss what she could do if there isn't a bin next to the toilet. What could she do instead?

- Encourage her to place a pad in her underwear and to walk around with it in place. Let her try the different types so that she can feel the differences between them.

- Try wearing a pad for the whole day, or even the weekend.

- Unwrap some tampons and tell her what they do and where you put them.

- Dip some tampons into water and see how quickly they absorb the liquid.

- Talk about the difference between tampons and pads. When is a good time for her to use a tampon?

- Share your own stories with your daughter – your first period, the products that you used, inserting your first tampon, how you felt, etc. Stories are important and your daughter will enjoy them.

- Discuss what she could do if she is out and doesn't have a pad. Who could she ask especially if she is at school? Show her how to fold up toilet paper to make up a temporary pad.

- Talk about how often she should change her pad, and how she can tell when it is due for a change. Let her know that it is normal for some blood to leak onto her underpants or sheets at night.

- Discuss where you will store products for her to use. Will she tell you if she runs out?
- Make up a period kit together and encourage her to keep it in her schoolbag.
- Talk about the importance of having clean hands when using pads, both before and after.

And don't forget to have fun. This doesn't have to be a formal teaching session. It is an opportunity for you to show your daughter that you are an expert and that she can come to you for advice.

Sexual feelings

During puberty, your daughter will experience sexual feelings for the first time in her life. The hormones that are busy making her body fertile are also making sure that she'll want to have sex so that she can become pregnant, which means that she will start to have sexual thoughts and be sexually attracted to either boys or girls.

It may help your daughter to know:

- During puberty, it is normal to become more aware of the opposite or same sex, and to feel more sexual.
- It is also normal to not experience sexual feelings. Asexuality is when someone is uninterested in sex or feels no desire for sex.
- Some girls will experience stronger or weaker sexual feelings than others. Some girls will start to have sexual feelings sooner or later than other girls. Everyone is different.
- In girls, the main physical sign of sexual excitement is wetness of the vagina. In boys, it is to have an erect penis.
- Sexual feelings can come from reading a romantic novel, watching a movie, or thinking about another boy or girl.
- Having sexual feelings is normal and is nothing to feel guilty about.

- Acting on such feelings with a partner is a big responsibility, and it is best to wait until older.

Masturbation

During puberty, your daughter might discover that touching or rubbing her clitoris and vulva can feel nice. Her vagina may become wet, moist, or tingly from self-stimulation, and she may experience orgasm.

An orgasm is a really nice feeling that can sometimes happen during masturbation or sexual activity. It is not easy to explain how an orgasm feels, because it can be different each time. You could describe it as a really nice feeling that starts in the genitals, and can also be felt throughout the whole body. This feeling then begins to feel stronger and stronger, building up until you begin to feel waves of intense feelings.

Masturbation is not harmful as long as it is kept private. There is no scientific evidence that it causes any harm to the body or mind. It is only a problem when it stops you from doing other things, or when it is done in public. However, there are many religious and cultural beliefs around masturbation.

It may help your daughter to know:

- Masturbation is often the first way girls can experience sexual pleasure.
- Many boys and girls begin to masturbate for sexual pleasure during puberty.
- Some boys and girls never masturbate. This is normal too.
- Masturbation does not cause physical or mental harm.
- Some cultures and religions oppose masturbation (talk to your religious leader).
- The decision about whether or not to masturbate is a personal one.
- Masturbation is a private activity.
- Many adults masturbate at some time in their lives.

Conception

Puberty happens for one reason – reproduction. This is so your daughter can become pregnant and start the next generation. She needs to know that this can happen and how it happens.

It may help your daughter to know:

- A baby is made when an egg from a female joins with sperm from a male.

- This can happen during sexual intercourse, when a man's penis is in a woman's vagina.

- Their bodies move together and after a short time, semen containing sperm comes out of the penis.

- The sperm travels up through the uterus and into the fallopian tubes. If one strong sperm joins with an egg, a baby begins to form.

- Babies can also be made with medical assistance, such as in vitro fertilization (IVF) or surrogacy.

Sex

Talking about puberty means also talking about sex. As puberty progresses, your daughter is going to start thinking of sex differently. Before puberty, she only thought of sex in a theoretical way, as something adults do. Now, as her hormones rewire her to reproduce, she will start to think of sex as something that she will want to do. This means you need to start talking to your daughter about sex. If you have never talked about sex with her before, don't expect her to be totally ignorant. It is very possible that she will have heard other kids talk about sex, or have read about it.

When talking to your daughter, it is important to remember that sex is more than the type of sexual activity that makes a baby. It can include oral sex, anal sex, and lots of touching where no penetration happens at all. Sex can also happen in lots of different ways. It might happen between two people who are in a loving and committed relationship, but it can also happen between two people who have only just met. Your daughter will hear a lot of mixed negative messages about sex and may need some help trying to interpret them.

When talking about sex, there are two parts to the conversation. First, it is about giving your daughter information, or the facts, for example, sex can be when the man puts his penis inside the woman's vagina. Second, it is about providing her with some guidelines about what is appropriate behavior, for example, you think she should wait until she is married, or in a loving, committed relationship, before she has sexual intercourse.

It is important that you tell your daughter what sexual attitudes and behaviors are okay, and not okay, in your family. And don't just tell her what they are. You need to explain why you feel this way, so your daughter can understand. Knowing the 'why' will help her while she is forming her own sexual values.

It may help your daughter to know:

- Sex can be lots of different things, but usually when you hear people talking about it, they are usually referring to sexual intercourse.

- Adults have sex for lots of different reasons:
  o To make a baby.
  o It feels good (it can also feel awful).
  o For fun.
  o It is a way to show love or to get close to someone.

- Sex is something that is just for adults. It isn't for kids and it isn't something that you should do with members of your family.

- Sex is something that is private and should only happen when … (share your beliefs about when it is okay for her to think about sex).

- Sex is special and is something that should happen with someone that you trust and care deeply about.

Consent

This is the age where you need to talk about consent in more detail. For the first time, your daughter is starting to explore what sex means. As you start to talk about sex, you also need to talk about consent for sex. Learning about consent will take many conversations.

It may help your daughter to know:

- Consent is when you agree to do something or you allow something to happen to you.

- In some situations, it isn't possible to give consent, such as when under the influence of drugs or alcohol.

- How to give or withhold consent and ask for it from others.

- How to seek help when she, or someone else, is having their right to consent violated.

- The consequences of not respecting consent, such as sexual assault, rape, or sex with a minor.

- Consent can be partial, for example, it is okay to do this but not this. 'You can kiss me, but don't put your hands down my shirt.'

- It is okay to change your mind later on, for example, you can withdraw consent at any time.

Same sex attraction

During puberty, your daughter will discover whether she is attracted to boys or girls. Some girls will already know this, but some won't have given it much thought until now. One in every 10 girls will be attracted to the same sex. It is possible that your daughter will be same-sex attracted. Who your daughter is attracted to is not her choice. She can't choose to like boys instead. It just isn't possible. She can try, but it won't work.

By now, she'll have already worked out that most girls like boys. It is what she sees on TV, reads about in books and sees around her. She will have also heard negative comments being made about gays, and she will have picked up on the fact that it isn't something that society as a whole is supportive about. Which means that for same-sex attracted girls, this can be a confusing time in which she will need your support. Whether you believe that same-sex attraction is okay or not okay, you still need to talk to your daughter about the fact that some kids are attracted to the same sex and not the opposite sex. All children need to know that sexual orientation is not a choice, that all people deserve respect regardless of their sexual orientation, and that who we are attracted to, whether it be boys or girls, is only a small part of who we are.

Just remember to discuss this topic with care and sensitivity, regardless of your beliefs. Sexual attraction is not a choice. If your daughter ends up being attracted to the same sex, how will she feel about it and will she feel safe talking to you about it?

It may help your daughter to know:

- Puberty is the time we usually discover which sex we are attracted to.

- She may feel attracted to the opposite or same sex. She may feel attracted to both sexes or she may not feel attracted to anyone. This is all normal.

- She will either like boys or girls, both or none. In time, she will know who she likes.

- She cannot change who she is attracted to.

- All people deserve respect regardless of their sexual orientation.

- Who we are attracted to, boys or girls, is only a small part of who we are.

- She needs to know about homophobia, and that some religions and cultures believe that same-sex attraction (homosexuality) is wrong.

Preventing pregnancy

Your daughter won't need a lot of information about contraception until she is showing an interest in boys or girls. You can give her the information, but it won't really be relevant until she is thinking about being sexually active. But she does still need to know that women can choose to prevent pregnancy.

It may help your daughter to know:

- When a man and a woman want to have sexual intercourse without having a child, they can use a family-planning method to prevent pregnancy.
- There are many types of family planning methods, also called contraceptives:
  - Abstinence, condom, implants, pill, injections, morning after pill.
- A girl cannot become pregnant if she has sex with another girl.
- Unprotected sex means having sexual intercourse without any contraception.
- Some religions and cultures are against the use of contraception.

Sexually transmitted infections (STIs)

Your daughter won't need a lot of information about STIs until she is showing an interest in boys or girls. You can give her the information, but it won't really be relevant until she is thinking about being sexually active. She does still need to know that there are infections that can be spread through sexual contact.

It may help your daughter to know:

- STIs are spread through sexual contact, which includes sexual intercourse and anal or oral contact. Some examples of STIs are:
  - Syphilis, gonorrhea, chlamydia, genital herpes, trichomoniasis, hepatitis B, human papilloma virus (HPV), and HIV.
- She can protect herself by using condoms and not having sexual contact with an infected person.
- STIs aren't nice things to have:

- o The symptoms for women can include genital sores or ulcers, lower abdominal pain or tenderness, unusual vaginal discharge, vaginal itching, painful urination, or painful sexual intercourse, depending on the STI.
- o The symptoms for men can include painful urination, urethral discharge, ulcers, or sores, depending on the STI.
- STIs need to be treated with medication or they can cause serious problems.
- Some STIs cause permanent infertility, chronic pain, and cancer of the cervix. Without treatment, heart and brain damage can develop 10-to-25 years after initial exposure to syphilis.
- Sex is not free of risks.

Online safety

As your daughter goes through puberty, she will become more curious about sex. She will also become more independent and not always come to you with her questions. Instead, she will head to the next best thing – the internet – to search for answers. She is going to stumble across sexually-explicit content – in the form of pornography – in her search for knowledge. She will also find information that looks reliable but isn't.

It may help your daughter to know:

- What your family rules are regarding the safe use of internet-enabled devices, as well as the consequences if she breaks these rules.
- Sometimes it is hard to tell if information on the internet is reliable or not.
- She will stumble across sexually-explicit images online (if she hasn't already). If she does, she should turn off the device and inform an adult that she trusts. Remind her that she won't get into trouble.

- Porn is not the best way to learn about sex. If she has any questions, she can ask you or find the answer in an age-appropriate book or website.

- Sending and receiving naked photos of private parts is illegal, until she is legally deemed an adult. The age varies in different countries but it is usually 16.

Boy changes

There are some boy changes that your daughter should also know about.

It may help your daughter to know:

- An erection is when the penis fills with blood and becomes hard and straight.

- Erections can happen when boys have sexy thoughts, or sometimes for no reason at all.

- Ejaculation is when semen comes out of a boy's erect penis when he is sexually excited.

- A wet dream is when his penis becomes erect, and he ejaculates when sleeping.

- Boys can't control when erections and wet dreams may happen.

- Ejaculation means that a boy is physically able to get a girl pregnant, if they have sexual intercourse.

How To
Talk About Puberty

*It isn't what you say that matters. What matters is that
you're giving your child the message that you're open to
talking to them about anything, no matter what.*

Getting started

The hardest part of talking to kids about puberty is getting
started. You know what you can talk about, but how do you
actually say it? How do you start the conversation?

It is normal to feel a little uncomfortable when you first start
talking about puberty with your daughter. We all do. Many of us
didn't have comfortable conversations with our own parents, growing
up. We don't have any helpful memories of what to do, just lots of
memories of what not to do! Like with all new things, it will get easier.
The more often you talk with your daughter about puberty, the easier
it will get.

You'll find many suggestions on different ways to start talking with
your daughter about puberty. Try to pick just one to start with, rather
than trying to do them all. Choose one that feels comfortable, or like

something you may already be doing. For example, if you already buy books for your daughter, buying a book on puberty is a great way to start.

Key messages

So, what are the main messages that you need to give your daughter?

- She isn't alone!
- You've been through puberty too, so you do understand what it may be like for her.
- She can talk to you about anything, no matter what.
- You will answer her questions truthfully.
- If you don't know the answer, you will find it and get back to her with it.
- What sexual attitudes and behaviors are okay, and not okay, in your family.
- She is normal!

At the end of the day, it isn't about how much information you share. It is about the fact that you are talking openly about growing up. This means that you will have an open relationship where your daughter can talk to you about anything, no matter what. As a parent, that is pretty much what we all want.

Everyday approach

The best approach with talking is to keep it as much like an everyday conversation as possible. If your daughter can sense a lecture coming on, she will tune out and stop listening almost immediately. Make sure you use an everyday tone and language. Try to talk about periods in the same voice and way that you would use when talking about her plans for the weekend. By sounding everyday (or natural), you are letting her know what is happening to her is normal and nothing to be ashamed of.

Get ready to repeat yourself, as you will need to have many conversations on the one topic before she will fully understand what you've been saying. This is completely normal and the way her brain works. Try to tell her a little bit more than you think she needs to know. As parents, we automatically tend to err on the side of caution and tell our kids less than they need to know, especially when it comes to love, sex and relationships.

Don't assume that she is too young or not ready for it. If she isn't ready, she'll just forget whatever it is that you said. When she is ready for that bit of information, she'll probably let you know.

Don't forget to listen, too. Listen to what she has to say, or what she thinks. She probably knows a lot more than you think she does.

When starting late

If you've never talked about any of this stuff before, it isn't too late to start, even if your daughter already has breasts, hair in new places or has started her period.

So, what's the best way to get started?

First, you need to warn your daughter that you are going to start talking about puberty and growing up. You could try explaining that you've realized that you haven't talked about puberty before, but that you would like to change that.

You could try saying:

- *A book I'm reading is about puberty. I know we haven't really talked about puberty before, but I'm going to try to change that, so we can have conversations about it.*

- *A book I'm reading made me realize how important it is for parents to talk with their kids about puberty. Since we haven't talked about it before, I'd like to start.*

Second, explain why you haven't talked to her about puberty and growing up before.

You could try saying:

- *It's something that my parents didn't talk about very much when I was a kid.*

- *I've always been worried that I would be bringing it up at the wrong time or the wrong place.*

- *I've always worried that I would get it all wrong or do as bad a job as my parents did.*

- *I've always been worried about saying too much or too little or even saying the wrong thing.*

- *Talking about sex makes me feel really uncomfortable.*

Third, explain what is going to change.

You could try saying:

- *I want us to be able to talk about anything, including sex. You are going to hear me talking about puberty and growing up. If you have any questions or want to talk about something, I want you to know that I am always available.*

Getting past your fears and worries

A lot of parents wonder if they are doing the right thing.

Maybe your daughter is too young for all this? Maybe or maybe not. Puberty happens whether kids are emotionally ready for it or not. Isn't it better that your daughter is prepared for the changes that will soon be happening to her, and for her to know that she can turn to you for support, guidance and information?

Won't you be encouraging her to be sexual? No, not at all. All you're doing is giving her information about what will be happening to her. You're also guiding her, because you're telling her what sexual behavior and attitudes are okay, and not okay, in your family. Research tells us that kids who have received good sex education are less likely to be sexually active and when they are, they will be much safer than their uneducated peers.[4]

She hasn't asked any questions yet, so maybe she isn't interested? Some girls ask questions and some don't. But it doesn't mean that she

---

4 SRE – the evidence. 2015. Evidence briefing. Sex Education Forum
http://www.sexeducationforum.org.uk/evidence.aspx

isn't interested. It just means that you will have to be the first one to bring it up.

Maybe you will say too much, or not enough? Or even the wrong thing? Possibly, but it doesn't really matter if you do. What matters is that you are showing your daughter that you are willing to talk to her about puberty, love, sex and relationships. You are letting her know that she can come and talk to you about anything. That's what really matters.

Getting comfortable with talking

It is normal for both parents and kids to feel uncomfortable talking about puberty. Luckily for you, it does get easier the more do it.

There are some things that you can do to help manage embarrassment:

- Let your daughter know if you sense that she is uncomfortable talking about puberty. Try saying:
  - *Some kids can feel really uncomfortable talking about puberty with their parents. I totally get it! I feel awkward talking about it too. Maybe we can help each other get past the awkwardness*

- Let your daughter know that you feel embarrassed. Try saying something like:
  - *I feel a bit uncomfortable talking about puberty because my parents never talked with me about it. But this is an important subject, so I really want to talk with you about it.*

- Keep it simple and talk about one topic at a time. Decide what you want to talk about, such as the need to wear deodorant to manage body odor. Spend a moment, and think about the best way to casually bring up the topic. You might say:
  - *Hey, I bought this for you at the supermarket today* (show her the deodorant). *Now that you're going through puberty, you'll sweat more and stink! This will help you to stink less. You just spray it onto each underarm. Just like this* (apply deodorant to yourself). *Does that make sense?*

- Talk when you're doing something else, such as washing dishes; this makes it seem like an everyday topic and not something to be ashamed of.

- Take a deep breath and take your time to respond to questions. There is no rush!

- Use humor. You don't have to make a joke about it, but laughing about puberty shows that it is a normal topic.

- Get some puberty books to read with your daughter. This way you don't have to stress about remembering what to say, as all the information is there in the book.

Sharing values

Don't forget to also talk about what sexual attitudes and behaviors are okay, and not okay, in your family. Don't just talk about the fact that you can prevent pregnancies with contraception. Share with your daughter what your thoughts are about contraception and unplanned pregnancy. Explain the reasons behind your belief so that your daughter understands why.

Don't just tell your daughter what sex is all about. Also let her know when you think it is a good time for her to think about sex. It might not be until she is married, or of legal age, or she must be in a loving, committed relationship first. Again, explain why, so that your daughter can understand the reasoning behind your beliefs.

Try to get into the habit of explaining what you think or believe when talking about love, sex and relationships. This is your opportunity to guide your daughter as she grows up, and to help her make healthy decisions around love, sex and relationships.

Share stories

Most kids are interested in hearing their parents' stories about growing up. Try to remember what it was like yourself, going through puberty. How did you feel? Who did you talk to? What were your fears? Sharing stories about what puberty was like for you reassures your daughter that you do know what she is going through. Plus, it is a great way to build connection and trust with your child.

Try saying things like:

- *I remember when I found my first pubic hair. I didn't know I would get hair down there, so I found some scissors and cut it off.*

- *I remember my first kiss. I really liked this person and one weekend at a party, we found a dark corner and kissed. All I really remember is this cold wet tongue being poked into my mouth, lots!*

- *I remember when I first started to like boys. I used to think about them all the time and daydream about being their girlfriend.*

- *I remember when my first period started. I was too embarrassed to say something to my mother. Right up until I left home, I used to sneak into her bedroom when she wasn't home and take one or two pads at a time.*

Take it slow

When talking to kids about puberty, there is no rush. Today, we know that the best way for kids to learn is through lots of frequent, repetitive conversations. If your daughter looks like she isn't listening, don't despair. She probably is listening, but she's hiding her discomfort by pretending not to. Keep on talking regardless. Just make sure you keep it conversational, don't turn it into a lecture and don't overdo it. Maybe keep it to one or two comments a week.

By keeping the conversation open, you are letting her know that she can come and talk to you about anything.

Be available

By talking to your daughter about puberty and growing up, you are letting her know that you are available and willing to talk. Make sure you tell her that she can come to you with any questions or concerns at any time. Don't be too pushy or obvious. You've got plenty of time to talk about all this stuff – there is no rush. If she throws you an opportunity to talk, make sure you grab it and talk. Yes, life does get busy, but five or 10 minutes of your time is often all that she needs.

Try to encourage her to talk about how she feels about growing up and changing. Ask her what she's looking forward to and what she's nervous about.

Normalize it

It is really important to normalize puberty for your daughter. She needs to know that what is happening to her is completely normal, and it is happening to her friends too.

It may help your daughter to know:

- Everyone is different.
- Some girls start early, some start late.
- Some girls develop fast, some develop slowly.
- Sometimes it can feel out of control.
- Going through puberty can be hard:
  o Your emotions swing.
  o Your body changes.
  o You start to have sexual feelings.
  o Your relationships with family and friends begins to change.
- Her body is doing what it is meant to do.

Indirect questions

Listen for indirect questions or disguised questions from your daughter. Some kids can be a bit vague and it may not be very clear what they are really asking about. Make sure you check back with your daughter and confirm that you have understood her question, and that you've given her enough information.

You could try saying:

- *Did that answer your question?*
- *Does that make sense?*

- *Was there anything else you wanted to know?*
- *Do you have any more questions?*

Find out what they already know

Kids can ask some very interesting questions. Sometimes though, there can be more than one answer, like the question, 'Where do I come from?'. There are many answers to this question – from hospital, my uterus, out of my vagina, from the apes. A good trick for working out what it is that your daughter is asking, is to ask her what she thinks. Instead of answering your question straight away, try asking her, 'What do you think?' This way, you can also work out what she already knows and just fill in the gaps.

Kids often dwell on a topic before they ask their questions, so she probably already knows the answer but just wants confirmation.

When you don't know the answer

Your daughter will ask you questions to which you don't know the answer. No one knows everything and I can guarantee that she is already asking you questions you don't have the answer for. The best way to manage this is to be completely honest and say, 'I don't know'. Then tell her that you'll find out and get back to her with an answer. If the topic isn't too risqué, you could both go and google it, or look it up in a book together. Just be careful when googling topics about puberty and sex, as you will often find pornography or content that isn't age-appropriate. Whatever you do, don't forget to get back to her with the answer. Forgetting could signal to your daughter that you aren't reliable, that the topic is taboo, or that you aren't comfortable answering these types of questions. This means that she'll start to look elsewhere for answers, which isn't a good thing.

Delaying answers

Sometimes, we just can't answer questions straight away. Your daughter may have asked you a question at the wrong time or the wrong place, or maybe you are just too busy or too uncomfortable to answer it on the spot. It is helpful if you can have your standard response to untimely questions worked out in advance. Acknowledge that she asked a question and explain when you'll respond.

You could try saying:

- *That's a great question, but how about we talk about that when we get home?*

- *I'm not sure about that. How about we talk about that later when I'm not so busy?*

- *You know what, I don't know. How about I find out the answer and I get back to you with it?*

If you get forgetful, send yourself an email, or post a note somewhere to remember. When you find the answer, you can restart the conversation with something as simple as, 'Remember how you asked me about periods earlier today? Well, I found the answer to your question'.

Third person

Talking in the third person can sometimes make it a bit less uncomfortable, for both you and your daughter.

You could try saying:

- *I saw your friend Amy the other day, and noticed that she's starting to grow breasts. It made me think that maybe we should be starting to talk about bras and things for when you start developing.*

- *One of the mums was talking today about how her daughter has started her period. It made me realize that we haven't really started to chat yet about periods.*

- *I heard a story on the radio today, where an expert was talking about how many girls don't understand what puberty is. Have any of your friends talked about puberty yet, or about any of the changes that are happening to them?*

Books

Books make talking about puberty a lot easier. There are a lot of puberty books that have been written specifically for girls. They'll provide your daughter with all the information she needs to know. You don't have to worry about trying to remember everything. Plus, the information in books is usually accurate, reliable, and written age-appropriately in language that our daughters will understand.

Some books are written for younger girls and will only talk about puberty and the changes that will happen. These books don't talk about sex, mainly because they target a younger audience, such as eight-to-11-year-old girls. There are also books that talk about puberty and growing up. Growing up always includes topics like love, sex, relationships, contraception, etc. These topics are always talked about in an age-appropriate way and are what 12-to-14-year-old girls are curious about.

Choosing the right book comes down to a number of things, such as the age of your daughter, her level of reading and how much information you are happy letting her have. If she is young, you'll want a book that won't overwhelm with too much detailed information, or talk about sex. You can get her a more detailed book later on.

Your instinct may be to go with a book that doesn't talk about love, sex and relationships. If she is really young (eight-10), or quite immature compared to her peers, that's fine. But do remember that you aren't protecting her by withholding information. If anything, you are leaving your daughter vulnerable, as she will just turn to her peers or the internet instead.

You can read the book together, or your daughter can have it to read alone. If she is reading it alone, just make sure that she knows that she can come to you with any questions.

You could try saying:

- *I heard about this great book on puberty so I bought a copy of it. We can read it together if you like.*

- *You've now reached an age where your body is going to start changing from being a kid to a grownup. I've bought a book that we can read together that talks about what will happen and why. How about we start reading it together tonight?*

- *Mary's mum told me about a book on puberty that she bought Mary to read. I bought you a copy to read by yourself, if you like. If you want to talk about anything in it with me, that would be great.*

To talk about the book later, you could try saying:

- *Remember how we read that book about puberty, well, I was wondering if you had any questions?*

- *Remember that puberty book I bought you? Well, I thought that maybe we should start to think about making up a period kit for you.*

To choose a puberty book you can visit your local library or bookshop. You will find a lot of puberty books listed and reviewed in this book review site: Sex Education Books for Children. (http://sexedrescue.com/sex-education-books-for-children/)

Answering personal questions

Your daughter may ask you some personal questions about puberty and sex that you won't feel comfortable answering. She might ask you about your first period, or about the first time you had sex. If the question is too personal, you don't need to answer it. See it as an opportunity to reinforce privacy but also try to turn it into an educational opportunity.

You could try saying:

- *That is a personal question that I'm not comfortable answering. But I know that it is illegal for children to have sex until they are 16.*

- *Some stuff is private and personal, so I don't really want to answer that question. But I know that they talk about that in your puberty book, so let's go and see what it has to say about it.*

Teachable moments

An easy way to provide information to your daughter is to find an everyday situation and turn it into an opportunity to teach something. At first you might find them a little bit hard to find. So, try thinking of one topic, for example, pornography, and start looking for opportunities to chat about porn. It could be a story on the radio, an article in the newspaper, a post that you found on Facebook, a blogpost, or something you read in a book. Once you start looking, you will find opportunities for talking, and teachable moments, everywhere.

Some opportunities for teachable moments could include:

- *Did you hear that story on the news about those teenage boys sharing videos of a drunk girl being raped? They are probably going to end up with a prison sentence for it. What do you think you would do if you were at a party and you saw your friends doing something like that? What could you do?*

- *See those two girls over there on the bench? The ones holding hands and kissing? How hard do you think it was for them to tell their family and friends that they were gay?*

- *Look at this magazine ad? Do you think that all women have bodies like that?*

- *Wow, did you hear the words to that song? It was about oral sex. They say that oral sex is something that teens often do with their first kiss? What do you think of that?*

- (Referring to a TV show or movie that you're both watching together) *Do you think that is right for that girl to have sex with her boyfriend because he says he will leave her if she doesn't?*

- *Can you put these tampons away for me in my bathroom? I guess that we should probably start talking about when you will get your first period. What do you think?*

- *Did you see what the ad on TV was about? It was talking about hair removal. You're going to start getting hair in some new places soon.*

Pre-warn them

If you want to talk about a particular topic, for example periods, let your daughter know in advance. It pre-warns her and can sometimes make her more receptive to talking.

You could try saying:

- *I want to talk to you this weekend about the different products that you can use for periods. It will be just you and me, with no other kids.*

- *I bought a puberty book for you today. I thought we could start reading it together before you go to bed tonight.*

- *Hey, I want to talk to you tonight about a sex/puberty thing. Don't worry, you're not in trouble or anything. I just want to talk.*

Conclusion

Congratulations! The fact that you have bought (and hopefully read) this book, means that your daughter is a fortunate girl! She is fortunate because she has a parent who:

- Wants to support her as she goes through a major phase of change in her life.

- Is someone she can turn to for the support, guidance and information that she needs, instead of turning to her friends or the internet.

- Wants to make sure that she has a better experience of puberty, than the one they had.

- Wants to talk openly with her about love, sex and relationships, even though sometimes it would be a lot easier to just avoid the topic.

- Is prepared to guide her as she works out what sexual behaviors and attitudes are okay and not okay, instead of leaving her to work it out on her own.

- Is now well prepared to start talking to her about puberty and sex, after reading this book.

So, keep this book as a resource that you can turn to when you need it. *Girl Puberty* will let you know the why, what, when and how of talking to your daughter about puberty.

And remember, it isn't so much *what* you say that matters, it is that you're talking to your daughter about growing up, and by talking, your relationship with her will grow stronger as she blossoms into a beautiful young woman.

Enjoy the journey!

Cath hak

Resources

Resources on puberty can be found at Sex Ed Rescue -
https://sexedrescue.com/resources/puberty/

Books for your daughter can be found at the Sex Ed Rescue book
review page, which is always being updated with new books -
http://sexedrescue.com/sex-education-books-for-children/

If you have questions to ask or want to connect with other parents
on the same journey, you can join my free parent Facebook group:
https://www.facebook.com/groups/thatparentgroup/

About the Author

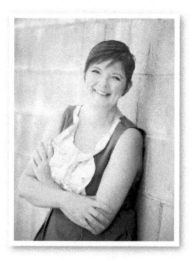

Cath Hakanson has been talking to clients about sex for the past 25 years as a nurse, midwife, sex therapist, researcher, blogger and educator. She's spent the past 10 years trying to unravel why parents (herself included) struggle with sex education. Her solution was to create Sex Ed Rescue, an online resource that simplifies sex education and helps parents to empower their children with the right information about sex, so kids can talk to them about anything, no matter what.

Cath has lived all over Australia but currently lives in Perth with her partner, 2 children, and ever-growing menagerie of pets. Despite having an unusual profession, she bakes, sews, and knits for sanity, collects sexual trivia, and tries really hard not to embarrass her children in public. Well, most of the time anyway!

If you'd like to know more, please visit my online home at
SexEdRescue.com

CPSIA information can be obtained
at www.ICGtesting.com
Printed in the USA
LVHW022342020521
686308LV00023B/834